VAGINAL ATROPHY

DOCTOR'S ADVICE ON HOW TO CURE VAGINA ATROPHY

DR. KATE .P

Contents

CHAPTER ONE

INTRODUCTION

The weakening, dryness, and inflammation of the vaginal walls caused by your body producing less estrogen is known as vaginal atrophy, also known as atrophic vaginitis. Vaginal atrophy can appear during breastfeeding or at any other time when your body's production of estrogen decreases, although it usually happens after menopause.

Vaginal atrophy causes pain during sexual activity for many women; if sex is difficult, you will naturally become less interested in it. Furthermore, there is a strong correlation between normal urinary system function and healthy genital function.

There are easy, efficient ways to treat vaginal atrophy. Your body will change as a result of lower estrogen levels, although vaginal shrinkage is not a permanent condition.

Symptoms

The following urine and vaginal signs and symptoms may be present in people with moderate to severe vaginal atrophy:

Dryness in the vagina

Burning in the vagina

discharge from the vagina

Vaginal itch

burning while passing gas

Urgency while voiding

An increase of UTIs

the inability to urinate

Light bleeding following sexual contact

discomfort during sexual activity

decreased lubrication of the vagina during
intercourse

vaginal canal shortening and tightness

When to visit a physician

Vaginal atrophy affects about half of postmenopausal women, according to some estimates, although few of them seek therapy. Many women accept the symptoms as part of who they are or feel too ashamed to talk about them with their doctor.

If you have vaginal symptoms such as unusual bleeding, discharge, burning, or soreness, or if you have painful intercourse that does not go away after using a vaginal moisturizer (Replens, Vagisil Feminine Moisturizer, etc.) or water-based lubricant (glycerin-free versions of Astroglide, K-Y Intrigue, etc.), schedule an appointment to see your doctor.

A reduction in estrogen production results in vaginal atrophy. Your vaginal tissues become thinner, drier, less elastic, and more delicate as your estrogen levels drop.

There could be a decrease in estrogen levels and vaginal atrophy:

following menopause

The years preceding menopause, or perimenopause,

While nursing

following the surgical menopause (surgical removal of both ovaries)

after cancerous pelvic radiation therapy

After cancer chemotherapy

As an adverse consequence of hormone therapy for breast cancer

Menopause-related vaginal atrophy may start to bother you in the years before menopause or may not become an issue until several years into menopause. Vaginal atrophy does not occur in all menopausal women, despite the condition being common. Having regular sex, whether with a partner or not, helps keep your vaginal tissues in good condition.

RISK ELEMENTS

Vaginal atrophy may be caused by a few things, including:

smoking. Smoking cigarettes impairs blood circulation, which deprives the vagina and other tissues of oxygen. Additionally, smoking lessens the effects of estrogens that are naturally present in your body. Furthermore, women who smoke usually go through the menopause earlier.

Not a single vaginal birth. It has been noted by researchers that women who have never given birth vaginally have a higher risk of developing vaginal atrophy compared to those who did.

Absence of sexual activity. Having sex, whether with a partner or not, improves blood flow and elasticity in your tissues.

Urinary tract infections and vaginal infections are more common in those with vaginal atrophy.

infections in the vagina. Your vagina's acid balance changes as a result of vaginal shrinkage, increasing your risk of developing a vaginal infection (vaginitis).

issues with the urine. Urinary atrophy, which is linked to atrophic vaginal alterations, is a condition that can lead to urinary tract abnormalities. Urinating more frequently, more urgently, or with burning could be experienced. Some females have higher rates of incontinence or UTIs.

CHAPTER TWO

Getting Ready for Your Consultation

Most likely, you'll start by talking to your primary care physician about your symptoms. Your primary care physician might suggest that you consult a gynecologist or internal medicine women's health specialist if you aren't already seeing one.

What you're capable of

In order to get ready for your appointment:

Jot down any symptoms or indicators that you're encountering. Even if they don't seem to be relevant to the purpose of your appointment, include them.

Important personal details should be noted. Add any significant strains or recent changes in your life.

Enumerate all prescribed drugs along with their dosages. Add all of the medications you use, including over-the-counter and prescription ones, vitamins, and supplements.

Think of bringing a friend or member of your family. It might occasionally be challenging to recall everything that was said during an appointment. It's possible that someone accompanying you will recall something you overlooked or forgot.

Get your questions ready. You only have so much time with your doctor, so you might maximize it by making a list of questions in advance.

Typical inquiries to make are as follows:

What is probably the root of my illness or symptoms?

What other factors could be causing my symptoms or condition?

Which tests are necessary for me?

Is my illness more likely to be acute or chronic?

Which line of action is the best one?

What are the alternatives you propose to the main strategy?

I also have a few additional medical issues. How do I oversee them both the best I can?

Are there any rules that I have to abide by?

Must I consult a specialist?

Are there any printed resources available to me, such as brochures? Which websites would you suggest?

Queries that your physician might pose

Your physician will inquire about your symptoms and perform a hormone status check. Your physician might inquire about the following:

What symptoms are you having with your vagina?

How long have these symptoms been bothering you?

Are you still having monthly periods?

To what extent are your symptoms bothering you?

Do you engage in sexual activity?

Does the illness restrict your sex life?

Have you received cancer treatment?

Do you take bubble baths or use scented soap?

Do you use feminine hygiene spray or are you a douche?

Which drugs, vitamins, and other supplements do you now take?

Have you used any lubricants or moisturizers available over-the-counter?

Vaginal atrophy diagnosis may include:

Pelvic exam: Your doctor will palpate your pelvic organs and visually inspect your cervix, vagina, and external genitalia during this procedure. Your doctor will also look for indications of pelvic organ prolapse during the pelvic exam, which include stretching of the uterine support tissues or bulges in the vaginal walls from pelvic organs like your bladder or rectum.

If you experience urinary symptoms, you should consider a urine test, which is gathering and evaluating your pee.

The acid balance test involves testing the acidity of your vagina by drawing blood from a sample or by inserting a paper indicator strip inside of it.

MEDICATIONS AND SUBTLES

Initially, your physician could advise that you:

To replenish moisture in your vaginal area, try using a vaginal moisturizer (Replens, Vagisil Feminine Moisturizer, etc.). It could be necessary for you to use the moisturizer every two to three days. In general, moisturizers have slightly longer-lasting benefits than lubricants.

To lessen discomfort during sexual activity, use a water-based lubricant (glycerin-free variants of Astroglide, K-Y Intrigue, etc.). Women who are sensitive to glycerin may feel burning and irritation, so look for products without this ingredient. If you use condoms as well, stay away from petroleum jelly and other petroleum-based items for lubrication. Upon touch, latex condoms can be broken down by petroleum.

Unpleasant symptoms that are not relieved by over-the-counter medications may benefit from:

topical estrogen in the vagina. The benefit of vaginal estrogen is that it works at lower dosages and exposes you to less estrogen overall because less of it enters your system. Additionally, it can offer more effective immediate symptom relief than oral estrogen.

estrogen taken orally. When you take estrogen orally, it enters your entire body. Ask your physician to go over the advantages and disadvantages of taking oral estrogen.

Topical estrogen

There are various variations of vaginal estrogen treatment. You can choose the one that works best for you and your doctor because they all seem to function equally well.

Cream for vaginal estrogen. Using an applicator, you immediately administer this cream into your vagina, usually before bed. How much cream to use and how often to administer it will be determined by your doctor. Women usually use it once a day for the first three weeks, and then once a week or three times a week after that. Creams can be messier than other kinds of vaginal estrogen, but they may also provide speedier relief.

ring of vaginal estrogen. A flexible, soft ring is inserted by you or your physician into the upper vagina. While in use, the ring releases a steady amount of estrogen and needs to be changed around every three months. The convenience this provides appeals to many women. Instead of being topical, a new, higher dose ring is regarded as a systemic treatment.

estrogen pill for vagina. You insert a vaginal estrogen tablet using a disposable applicator. How often to insert the tablet will be explained to you by your doctor. For example, you could use it twice a week after the first two weeks of daily use.

Estrogen treatment administered systemically

In cases where vaginal dryness is accompanied by additional menopausal symptoms, such intense or moderate hot flashes, your doctor can recommend using progestin and estrogen pills, patches, or gels, or a higher dosage estrogen ring.

Although combination estrogen-progestin patches are also available, progestin is often administered as a tablet. Discuss with your physician the pros and cons of hormone treatment based on your medical condition as well as any family medical history.

Alternative treatments

Because of worries that even low levels of estrogen may eventually raise the risk of endometrial and breast cancer, researchers are trying to identify alternative treatments for vaginal atrophy.

Inform your physician whether you have ever had breast cancer, and take into account the following:

therapies without hormones. First, try using lubricants and moisturizers.

estrogen in the vagina. If nonhormonal therapy are ineffective for your symptoms, your doctor may suggest low-dose vaginal estrogen in collaboration with your oncologist. Vaginal estrogen may, however, raise your chance of the cancer returning, particularly if your breast cancer was hormone-sensitive.

estrogen treatment administered systemically. In general, systemic estrogen treatment is not advised, particularly if your breast cancer was hormone-sensitive.

WAY OF LIFE AND DOMESTIC MEDICINE

Sexual engagement on a regular basis, with or without a partner, may help avoid vaginal atrophy. Blood flow to the vagina is increased during sexual activity, which supports the health of the vaginal tissues.

OTHER FORM OF MEDICINE

Menopause-related vaginal dryness and irritation are treated with certain alternative medications, however few of these methods have clinical trial data to support them. The field of complementary and alternative medicine is gaining popularity, and scientists are attempting to weigh the advantages and disadvantages of different supplementary therapies for vaginal atrophy.

Before using any food or herbal supplements for menopausal or perimenopausal symptoms, consult your doctor. Herbal drugs can be hazardous or interfere with other medications you take, endangering your health. The Food and Drug Administration does not regulate these items.

THE END

www.ingramcontent.com/pod-product-compliance
Lightning Source LLC
Chambersburg PA
CBHW061930270726
48660CB00003BA/1121